AROMATHERAPY FOR BEGINNERS

PRACTICE YOUR OWN WELL BEING through HOLISTIC HEALING

Disclaimer

What You Will Find In This Book?

One of nature's many gifts can easily and readily be accessible through aromatherapy. It is not a practice for hippies and new agers. Anyone can try out the many benefits of this practice with **Aromatherapy for Beginners**.

Aromatherapy makes use of precious natural elements that are ethically framed and pose no adversity if used correctly. For the well-being of your physical and psychological health aromatherapy may just be the way to the greater goodness that your body needs.

Read on if you are curious to try out the wonders of including this pleasurable practice in your lifestyle.

The **Aromatherapy for Beginners** contains the following:

1. A comprehensive introduction to the practice of aromatherapy.
2. Authentic Intel on essential oils.
3. Aromatherapy recipes by the benefit you are seeking.
4. Various Aromatherapy products.
5. Proven Benefits of Aromatherapy.

So just go ahead, flip the page and try out a few to experience the real Aromatherapy benefits!

Contents

The Lead In To Aromatherapy

Aromatherapy is dedicated to the wellbeing of two things: your physical and your psychological well-being. It is done by first extracting the natural oils from flowers roots, stems and bark or any other part of a plant.

Many consider Aromatherapy to be a form of substitute medicine. It involves you inhaling essential oils, either that or you could have a massage where the oils travel through your skin into the blood stream. The inhaling stimulates brain function while the skin absorption boosts the body's healing power.

Essential Oils are the pure essence of the plant you choose for the extraction. The name 'Essential Oils' is simply coined in to categorize all those aromatic and natural plant oils that have CO_2s and absolutes incorporated.

However the use of essential oils only I not the restriction applied to aromatherapy. The practice can also be done with other organic material like mud, clays, sugars, sea salts, milk powders, herbs, hydrosols, liquid wax jojoba and vegetable oils (cold pressed).

Essential Oils

Essential oils come from the term quintessential oil. Quintessential oils come from the Aristolean time when it was believed that everything is created from any of the 4 elements namely water, earth, fire and air. The fifth element was believed to be quintessence. Quintessence is the life force of a living being. The process of distillation and evaporation were believed to take out the 'spirit' or the life force from the plant, thus the word quintessential oil. However, we know that essential oils are not 'spirits' but actual tangible mixture of chemicals.

For an oil to be an authentic essential oil it has to be separated by physical means like distillation or cold pressing.

Since Essential oils are made up of pure essences it is obvious that these are concentrated in nature for 1 drop of essential oil is enough to make 30 cups of herbal tea. This goes to guide that essential oils must never b use without a carrier oil.

Benefits of Essential Oils

Widely essential oils are used either to cure or relieve the body of a problem like stress or headache. Let's look at the various organic essential oils by the problems they solve.

Essential Oils to Use For Stress:

Rosemary

Palmarosa

Ylang Ylang

Sandalwood

Melissa

Cedar wood

Frankincense

Rose

Clary Sage

Jasmine

Neroli

Bergamot

Chamomile

Lavender

For Insomnia use the Essential Oils:

Cedar Wood

Marjoram

Geranium

Bergamot

Neroli

Chamomile

Rose

Lavender

Essential Oils Used For Anxiety:

Sandal wood

Rosewood

Neroli

Marjoram Geranium

Lavender

Basil Bergamot

Essential Oils Used For Wounds and Cuts:

Thyme

Oregano

Bergamot

Lemon

Geranium

Eucalyptus

Tea Tree

Lavender

Essential Oils Used For Constipation:

Rosemary

Lemongrass

Black Pepper

Anise

Fennel

Essential Oils Used For PMS:

Ylang Ylang

Rosemary

Rose

Melissa Neroli

Lavender

Juniper Berry

Geranium

Sweet Fennel

Clary Sage

Chamomile

Bergamot

Essential Oils Used For Headaches:

Thyme

Rosemary

Melissa

Marjoram

Lavender

Peppermint

Eucalyptus

Clary Sage

Chamomile

Cajeput

Essential Oil Synergy is what one calls a specific blend of essential oils for their specific therapeutic purposes. A synergistic blend is believed to be more effective if you have a certain benefit in mind for the aromatherapy you are taking. Many experts believe in doing this instead of blending the essential oils to produce appealing and complicated aromas.

Hydrosols

Also more commonly known as hydrolats is the water that results after distillation. They harbor water-soluble parts of a plant and the microscopic components of essential oils. Every liter of hydrosol contains less than a percent of dissolved essential oils. Hydrosols also have carboxylic acids which is the primary reason for their anti-flammatory properties.

The proper way to store hydrosols is by placing them in the refrigerator. They last from around 12 months to up to 2 years.

Hydrosols work to benefit the skin and thus are found in many skin care products especially cleansers and creams. Some of their benefits are healing wounds and cuts, cooling the skin (anti-flammatory), incorporated in toners they increase effectiveness and they are also very good as hydrating agents in various skin products.

German Chamomile scientifically known as Matricaria Recutia is a hydrosol that works best as an anti inflammatory product. Its cooling properties are used to treat eczema, acne, rashes and psoriasis.

There are several other commonly used and effective hydrosols like Clary Sage scientifically known as Salvia Sclarea. This hydrosol works as a great anti depressant and is commonly used for PMS and hot flashes.

Another hydrolat is the beautiful scented Lavender also known as Lavandula Angustifolia. It is used for its relaxing properties and in baths or as a spritzer.

Orange Flower is what people call the Neroli is a hydrolat used for stress relieving and an all rounder for skin care. It is scientifically known as Citrus aurantium var. amara.

Witch Hazel is used as a cut, wound, insect bite cleanser; also used for acne and oily skin. It is scientifically known as Hamamelis Virginiana.

Basic Essential Oils to Have On Hand

Aside from the oils that pose their designated benefits you must have certain essential oils all the time on hand. Most of the essential oils have common benefits so the wisest thing to do would be to choose the ones that you need.

Lavender is a must have. You can use it to make your own homemade mouthwash, eye lotion and skin tonic. It has significant stress relieving and relaxation qualities and is great for avoiding rheumatism, arthritis and scars. It is used as a cure for many skin disorders due to its prompt healing process.

There is little wonder in the fact that in Germany Chamomile is known as alles zutruat which translates into "capable of anything', Chamomile oil is an effective soother for toothaches, abscesses, neuralgia, earache, bruises, burns, allergies, inflammation, fever, cramps and digestive problems.

Bergamot oil can only be used in its diluted form. It is used for scalp conditions and for dressing skin wounds. Deodorants and breath fresheners are made from Bergamot oil and its most favorable quality is the ability in the oil to lower anxiety and depression. Bergamot is used in aromatherapy to boost the aroma of several other mixtures that are to be used in the treatment.

Tea Tree Oil is great for its anti-septic qualities. It helps with tons of things like sore throats, head lice, thrush, allergic break outs, acne and abrasions. Tea Tree oil is widely famous for its anti-septic properties. Plus many homeowners use it in household cleaners to avoid the extreme chemicals that are used in cleaners with bleach.

Eucalyptus is great as an inhalant for respiratory issues. The oil is used to heal skin irritations, fever reduction, insect bites and also for the purpose of disinfecting the air.

Does It Really Work?

Many a time's people have wondered if aroma therapy can cure major problems like some psychological diseases. This is due to word 'cure' associated with aromatherapy in many journalistic fluff pieces. In the United States there is no law that governs and restricts the use of the word aromatherapy to its authentic practice. This has allowed many manufacturers to slap on the word aromatherapy into everything they deem fit.

Aromatherapy is an age old practice. An indicator of unreliable claims is when manufacturers advertise it as a new thing or an amazing new find. Aromatherapy has been around for years.

Holistic aromatherapy does not require the use of fragrance oils or any synthetic product. Fragrance oils used in aromatherapeutic candles exhaust toxins when the candle is burned.

Aromatherapy relives depression and stress but does make you immune to it permanently. Aromatherapy was never intended to be an alternative to the standard medicine. Keep a realistic mindset and you will see how aromatherapy alleviates your mood, eliminate stress and makes up for an overall beneficial experience.

Aroma therapy has incredibly valid and exquisite uses for the human body. It is important that you educate yourself when it comes to the different essential oils and their specific benefits.

However never fall prey to claims that aromatherapy is a miracle worker and should not be depended upon as a cure but once you introduce aroma therapy into your lifestyle you will experience improvement.

The Natural Science of Aroma Therapy

Aromatherapy makes use of various natural occurring essential oils. It is the unique qualities of the essential oils that are transferred to the human body for their benefits. The essential oils are extracted from the plant by the two methods: distillation and expression. S Within the view of holistic aromatherapy essential oils are considered harmful for handling and come with their own set of safety instructions that need following. It does not matter how nice they smell they must be handled with great care.

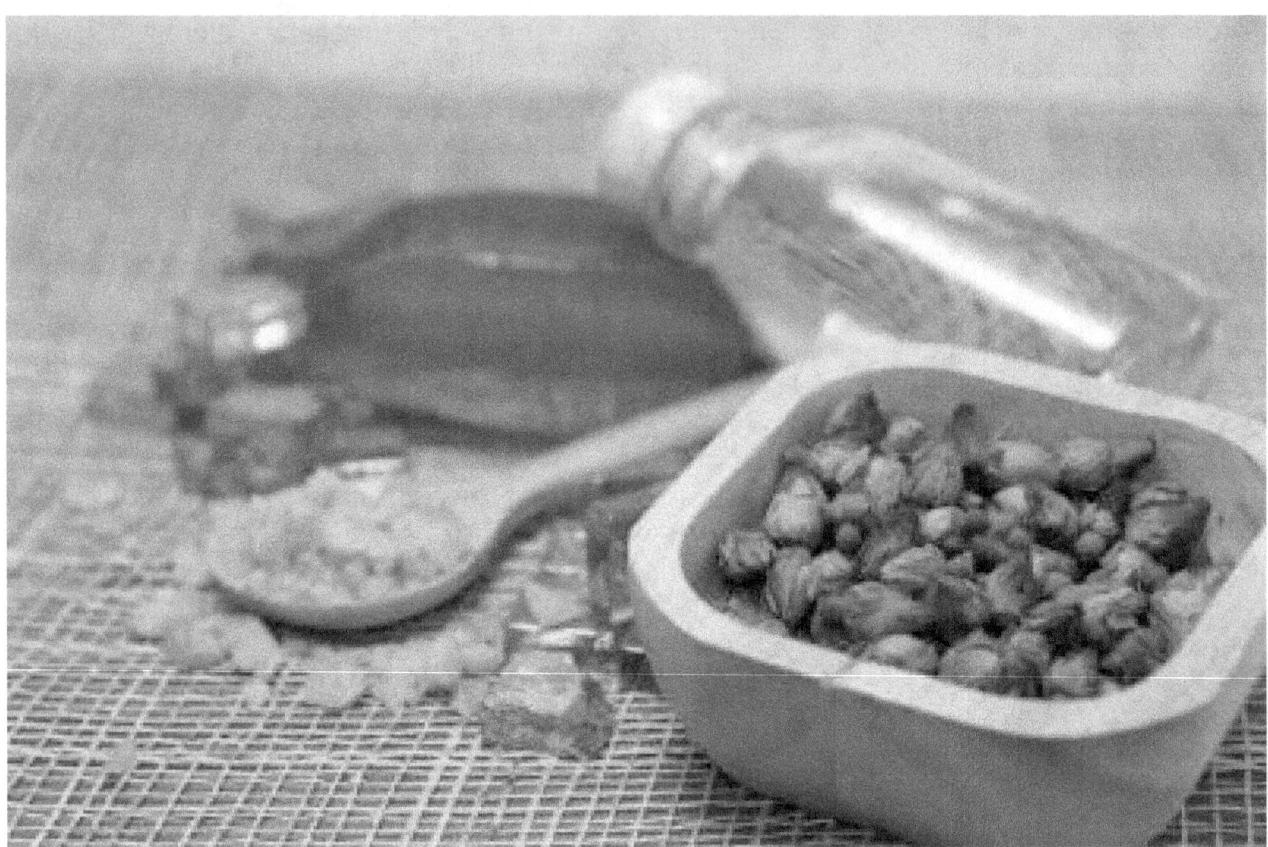

To Use Or Not To Use

Many companies and manufacturers claim that their labels must be used till the full strength for the best results and effect. The truth is that first off essential oils should not even be used undiluted. Secondly they cause permanent sensitization when used in full strength, unless of course the product you have at hand has synthetic components. Moreover, it is a common speculation that companies that instruct their customer to us the essential oil in its full strength instead of the little droplets that are recommended are actually doing that in hopes of the customer using up the products quickly and you would have to buy more.

Safety Precautions

Essential oils are a pure essence and thus are extremely concentrated products. The safety precautions highlighted below are a great

Essential Oils are never to be used on the skin undiluted. A lot of labels for oils advertise otherwise and many aromatherapy practitioners make exceptions for example everyone thinks that lavender and tea tree oil are not that harmful they can be used undiluted and they do so, however it has been noticed that these two can still cause reactions to sensitive skin.

If you come across oil that you have never used in your life before it's a much safer option if you try a skin patch test first for hat specific oil. Certain oils used in aromatherapy can cause allergic reaction and sensitization to certain skin types. So it's safer if you know firsthand which oil is for you and which Is not.

Certain conditions exclude the people from having an aromatherapy. Even though its true whatever benefits aromatherapy provides however the strength and properties of the essential oils in use might cause an adverse effect which however not proven are much wiser to stay away from. If you have epilepsy, asthma or are pregnant it's better to consult the essential oils profile before you choose the blend for yourself.

Just because one drop of essential oil is doing a great job does not mean that two will double the benefit. Stick to lower quantities. Remember that less is more when it comes to essential oils in aromatherapy. Using a higher proportion of the essential oil blend might ruin the entire aromatherapy.

Here is a mistake that people make all the time. Not all essential oils listed in existence are meant for use in aromatherapy and certain essential oils are only safe when handled by experts or highly experienced practitioners of aromatherapy. For example, sassafras, bitter almond, rue, wintergreen, horseradish, camphor, onion, pennyroyal and Wormwood.

Never allow children near essential oils. Or better yet store your essential oils somewhere away from the reach of little kids. Many essential oils have an amazing smell and certain even smell edible and safe to drink such as the citrus oils. No matter how appealing embed in your mind that all oils are poison.

An important thing that must be addressed is that though essential oils are blended or aromatherapy which has the individual inhaling these, you must not and should never consume any essential oils as they are out of the bottle. In fact they should not even be tasted. There are circumstances when essential oils are internally taken but that is after a conformed and detailed prescription of a highly qualified aromatherapy practitioner.

Essential Oils are extremely flammable so when you are planning to keep them away from the reach of children, make sure they are well away from any sparks pr potential fire hazards.

The Skin Patch Test

Many experts claim that most of the hydrosols are safe to use once they are undiluted. However better safe than sorry; it is incredibly vital that one performs a skin patch test for every hydrosol in use.

Step 1

Start by placing no more than 2 drops of essential oils on your elbow. It is not wise o apply undiluted essential oils directly on your skin.

Step 2

Next make sure that you don't get this area of application wet or in contact in water. Now stick a bandage to this part of the skin.

Step 3

This is the most important step. If after applying the bandage you feel irritation or experience any sort of reaction to the skin, don't waste any time and remove the nbadage and wash that area gently and thoroughly with water and mild soap.

Step 4

However, if the effect is the opposite of what is described in step 3; in other words if there is no adverse reaction or irritation to the skin in the following 24 hours you must acknowledge that the essential oil when diluted is safe for your skin.

Keep In Mind That...

If a certain essential oil is not bad for you must be aware that it could be a factor for allergy for others. So be careful and keep your essential oil collection away fro direct skin contact.

Moreover, you must automatically know which diluted essential oils not to try the patch test on because if you are allergic to a certain plant chances are you will be allergic to

its essence too.

How to Dilute Essential Oils Before Using In Aromatherapy

Using essential oil on skin without first diluting them with carrier oil is said to applying them as neat. Let's be first clear on rule number one on aromatherapy essential oils: Never apply essential oils without diluting them first!

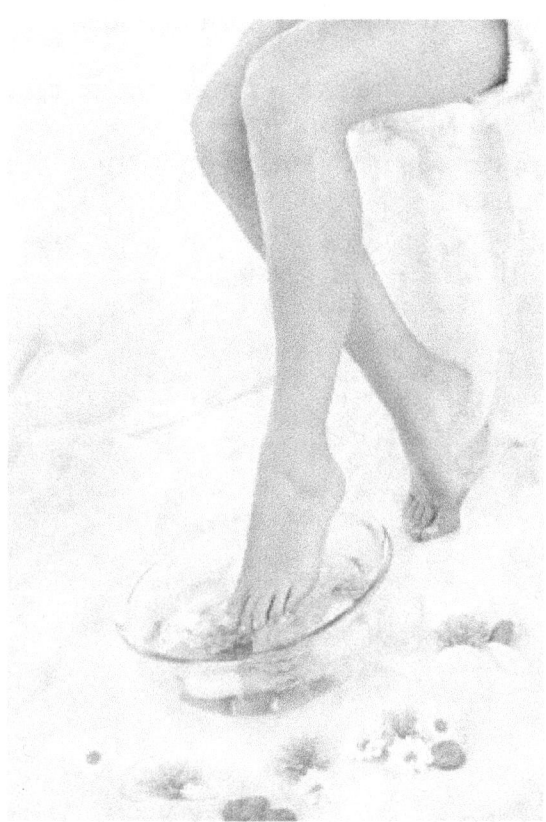

Many expert aromatherapy practitioners do this however it should be avoided at all costs. Repeat the mantra "sensitization forever'. For example though a lot of people use lavender oil without any adverse reaction but when you apply it n cracked skin you are in a for a surprise. Plus diluting the essential oils are not only good for you but also save on cash.

Everyone has a different skin type so the reaction to essential oils are varied too.

Sensitization

Sensitization occurs in the form of a skin rash or allergy although the symptoms of this are different for everyone. Sometimes it is severe and sometimes it just feels itchy. The unfortunate thing about this is that once you get sensitized because of an essential oil it is very much likely that you will be sensitized by that oil forever no matter how many times you try it again by diluting it first. Nevertheless, sensitization should not be taken lightly. There can be severe cases for this too like anaphylactic shock and several respiratory problems. Once you experience an adverse reaction or sensitization to an essential oil it increases the potential for you to experience an adverse reaction from other essential oils and the products that harbor these oils.

Essential oils demand to be treated with great care and gentleness. The safety measures outlined in this book are not meant to scare you from using these, just to warn you about the consequences of mishandling them. If handled with the proper way essential oils are quite harmless.

Essential Oil Dilution for Topical Application

Using essential oils for topical use takes up only 2% oil dilution. However for the elderly and little children your dilution must be cut to 1%. Aromatherapy makes us e of separate essential oils for children. Do not make use of the oils that are not suitable for children.

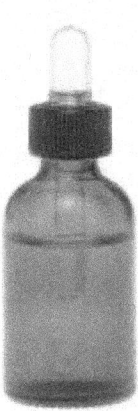

Here is something that you must keep in mind when you diluting the essential oil yourself. Today many people are accustomed to synthetic fragrances that are everywhere in all skin products like creams, lotions and soaps. Your sense of smell may be accustomed to a much stronger sense of smell than the diluted essential oil will smell like. You might not even notice the aroma of the essential oil for some time first. Ensure that you are not over doing the proportions in a blend.

The Easy Guide To Making The 2 % Dilution Without Overdoing It

A good strategy is to put only 12 drops of essential oil in an Oz of carrier oil. That's 30 ml of cold pressed carrier oil. You can alternate this with an organic moisturizer, vegetable butter and lotion.

In reality there is no best way to measure the 2 % of the essential oils. Experts claim that the easiest way is to measure by the drop but un luckily there is no standard drop size because the temperature of the oil may vary, dropper size or the orifice reducer. However this method works for making topical blends but in small quantities.

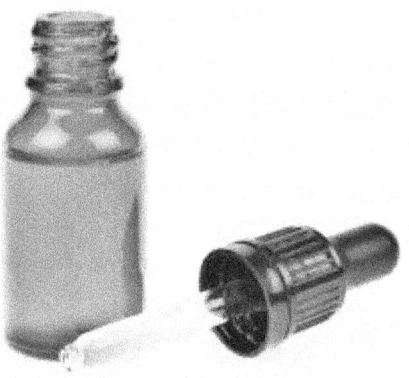

A common practice like the raindrop therapy involves applying pure and undiluted essential oils in to the skin without any mixing with carriers. This leads to skin burning and is quite painful. A lot of practitioners promote this as the 'toxins exiting the human body'. It is important to acknowledge that authentic aromatherapy does not claim any crude generalizations. The reason to outline this is to remind the readers the consequences of this.

Shopping For Aromatherapy Products 101

Product labeling and ingredients description deserve the attention when it comes to aromatherapy products.

When it comes to the marketing claims remember that 'aromatherapy' is a buzzword. What is more, in The United States there are zero regulations for this, which gives many companies the perfect opportunity to exploit the term aromatherapy and sell products that have nothing to do with the authentic aromatherapy. So a word to the wise, be careful.

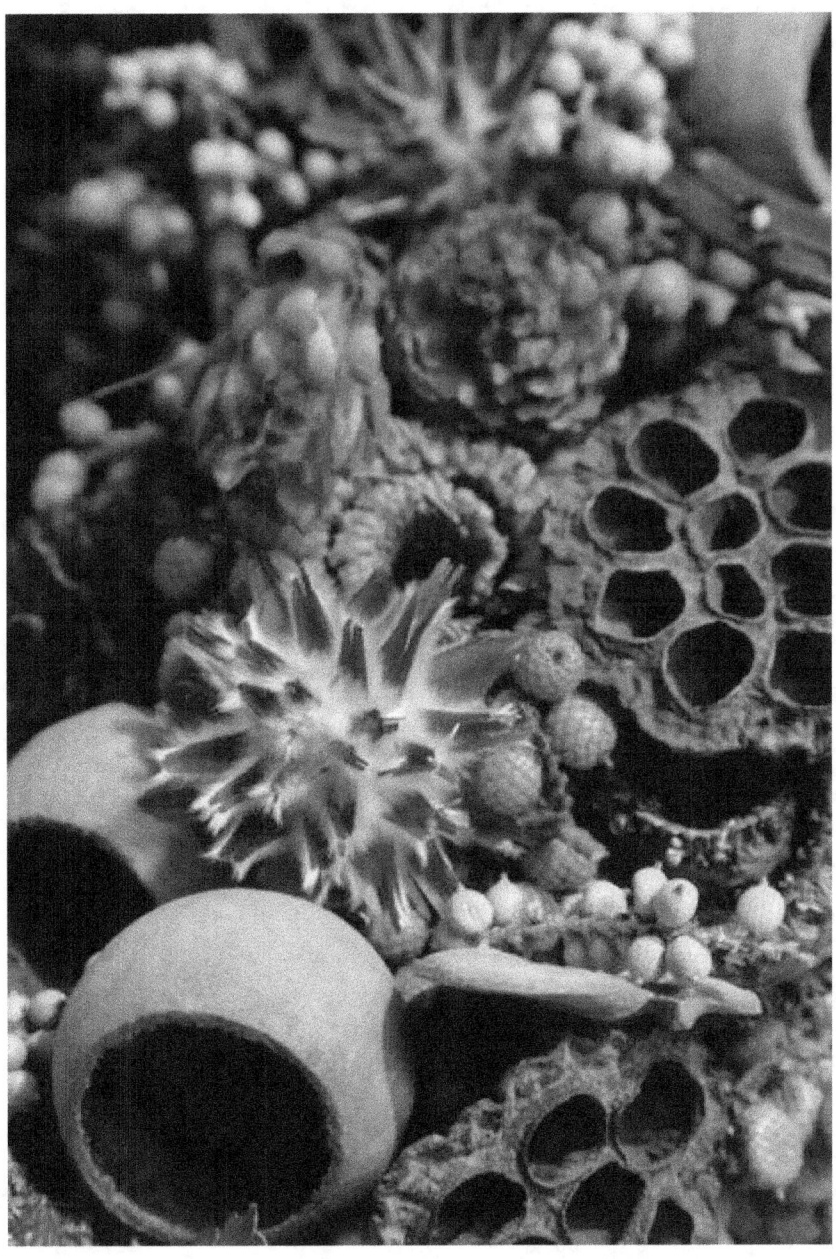

Here is what you need to do.

Tip 1: Read the Ingredients label

Go through the ingredients and mentally categorize the synthetic ingredients and the natural ones separately. Now remember to look out for the ingredients that you think are hazardous or are not suitable for your skin type.

However if a product does not list the list of ingredients just switch to another label without a backward glance. Here the fortunate aspect of shopping for aromatherapy products: authentic aromatherapy product sellers are aware of the fact that serious aromatherapy practitioners want to know what is exactly inside the products they are buying and readily provide the natural ingredients list. But this back fores too, certain authentic manufacturers are afraid that their blends might be stolen by other companies. As it is the aromatic formulas that are most precious.

Tip 2: Do Your Homework

Where ever and whoever you plan to purchase from make sure you make the effort to learn whatever you can about them. Most companies have detailed websites for their customer's disposal. This is an easy step as most reputable companies that supply aromatherapy products state their company history, affiliations and educational background.

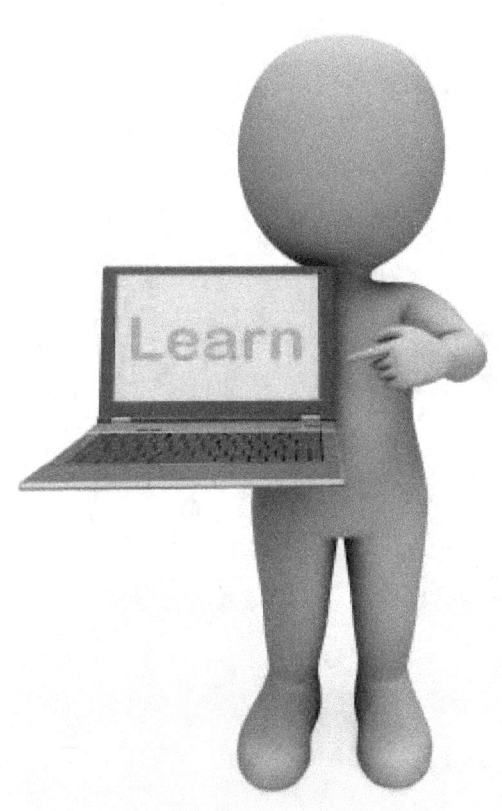

Tip 3: Be Cautioned

Companies that do not focus on all 100% natural ingredients always sound fishy. It is best if you stay away from this sort. This leads to our next tip.

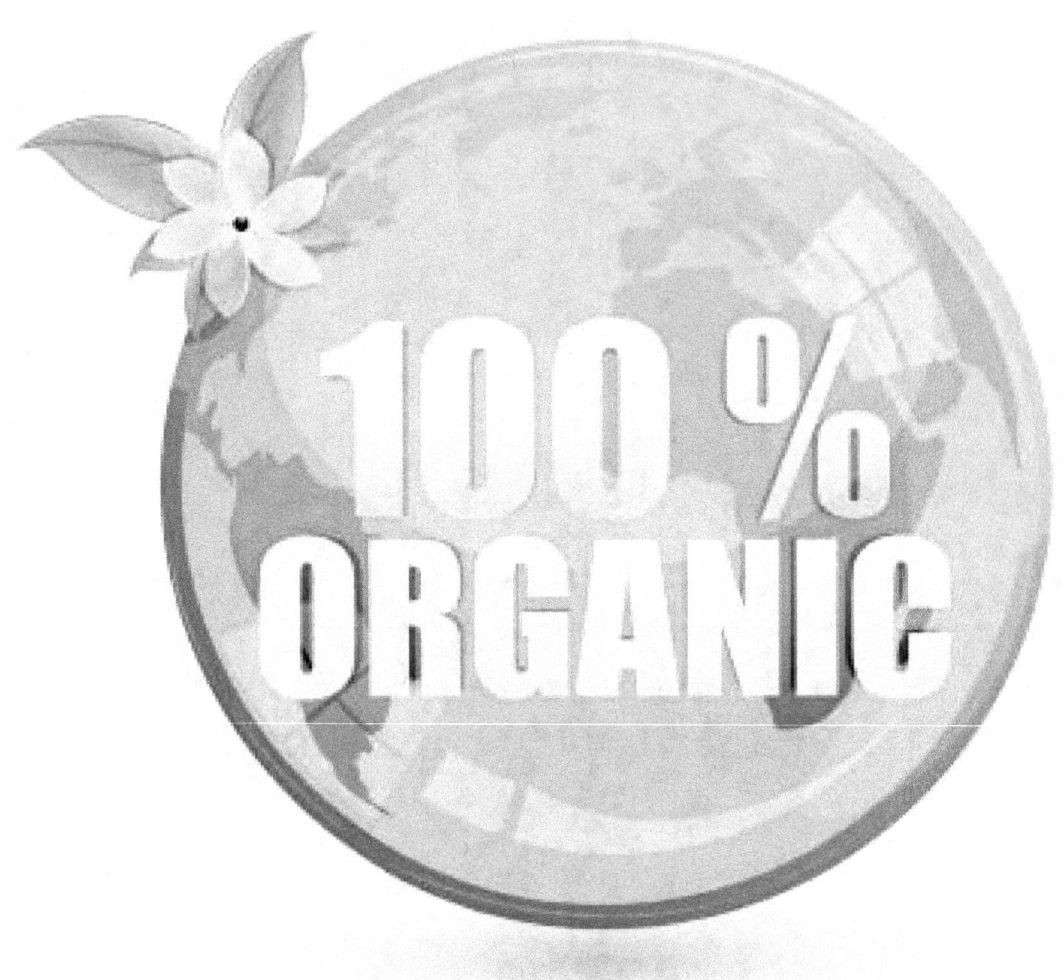

Tip 4: The Marketing Hype

No law can stop the companies from advertising their products as MADE FROM ESSENTIAL OILS or FORMULATED FROM NATURAL INGREDIENTS. What we as buyers miss out easily is that it does not claim that is 100% made out of natural ingredients. Such marketing jibes have us buying products that incorporate synthetic ingredients with a very small amount of the natural ingredients.

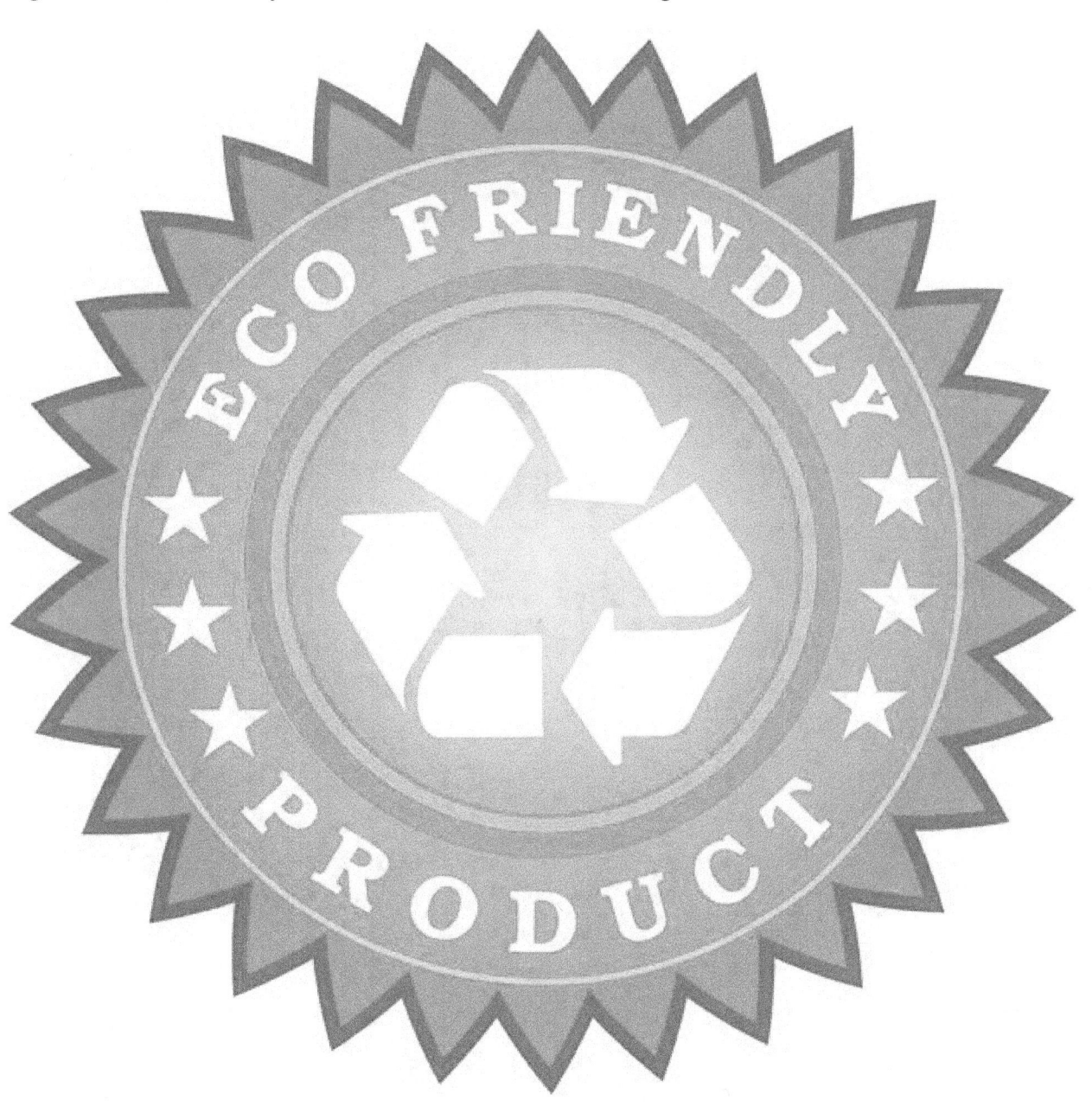

Tip 5: There Are Products That Rightly Say 100% Natural

When you are confused with two of the same products with different companies and both of them have 'natural ingredients' in them. Buy the one that says all natural ingredients.

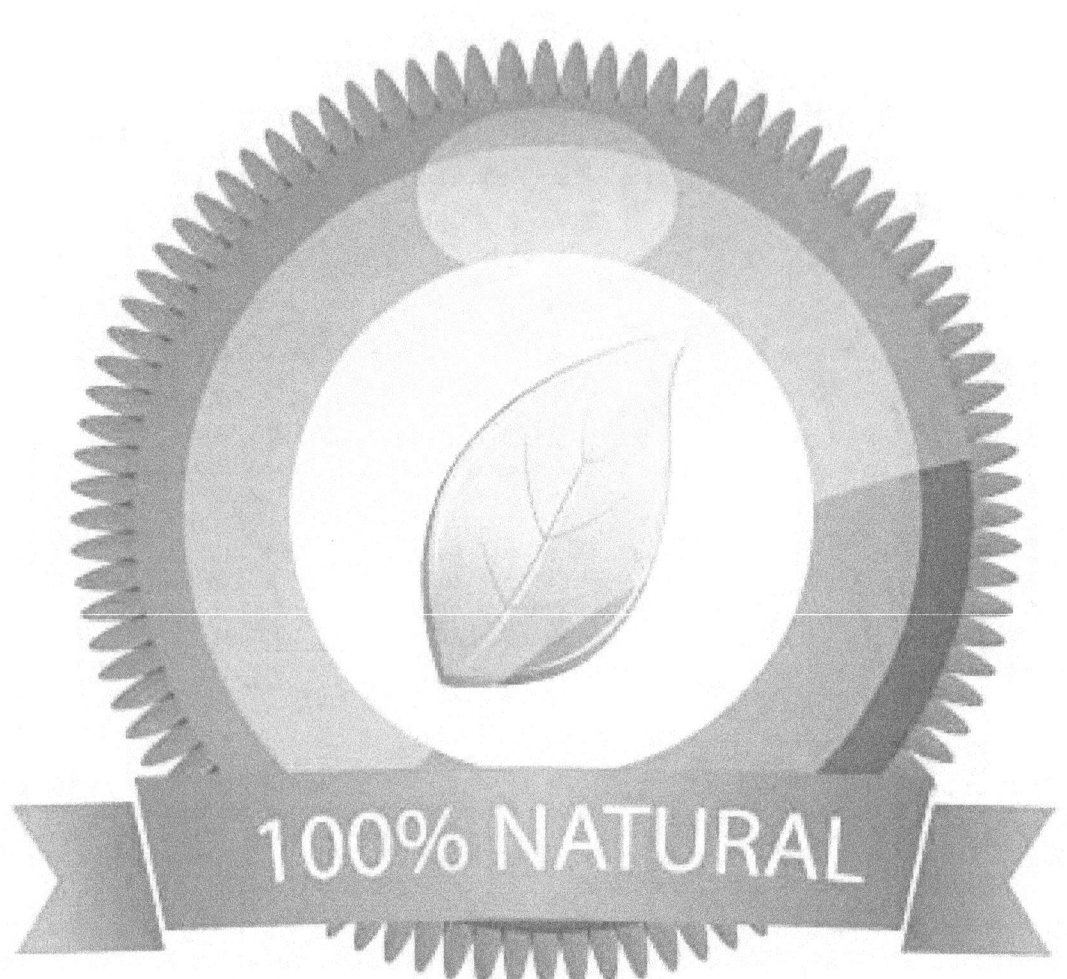

Aromatherapy Recipe Blends- By The Use

Body Massage Oil Recipe

When making your own diffuser blend remember to use the recipes below by increasing each quantity four times and mixing the blend and storing it in a dark colored glass bottle.

If you want to use the blends via air freshener than increase your blends ingredient quantity 6 times what it is. You should have a final count of 30 drops. Use this in the standard Mist Recipe below.

Mix the essential oil blend of your choice in an Oz of carrier oil of your choice (olive oil. Almond oil, coconut oil).

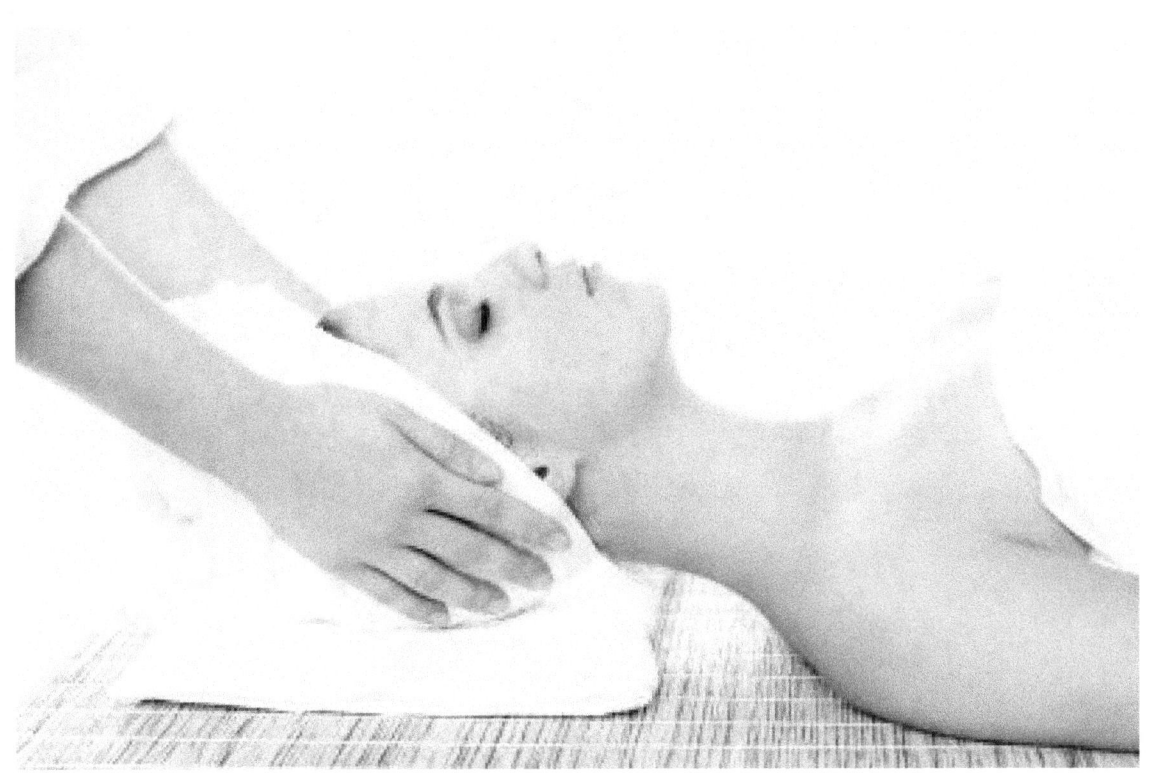

Mist Recipe

Aromatherapy blends work miracles for massages. Just multiply the ingredient quantity by two, make sure the total drops are 10 and then use your blend of choice in The Body Massage Oil recipe below.

Use 3 Oz of steam distilled water into a spray bottle and then add the 30 or 40 drops of essential oil blend. Shake the bottle every time before use.

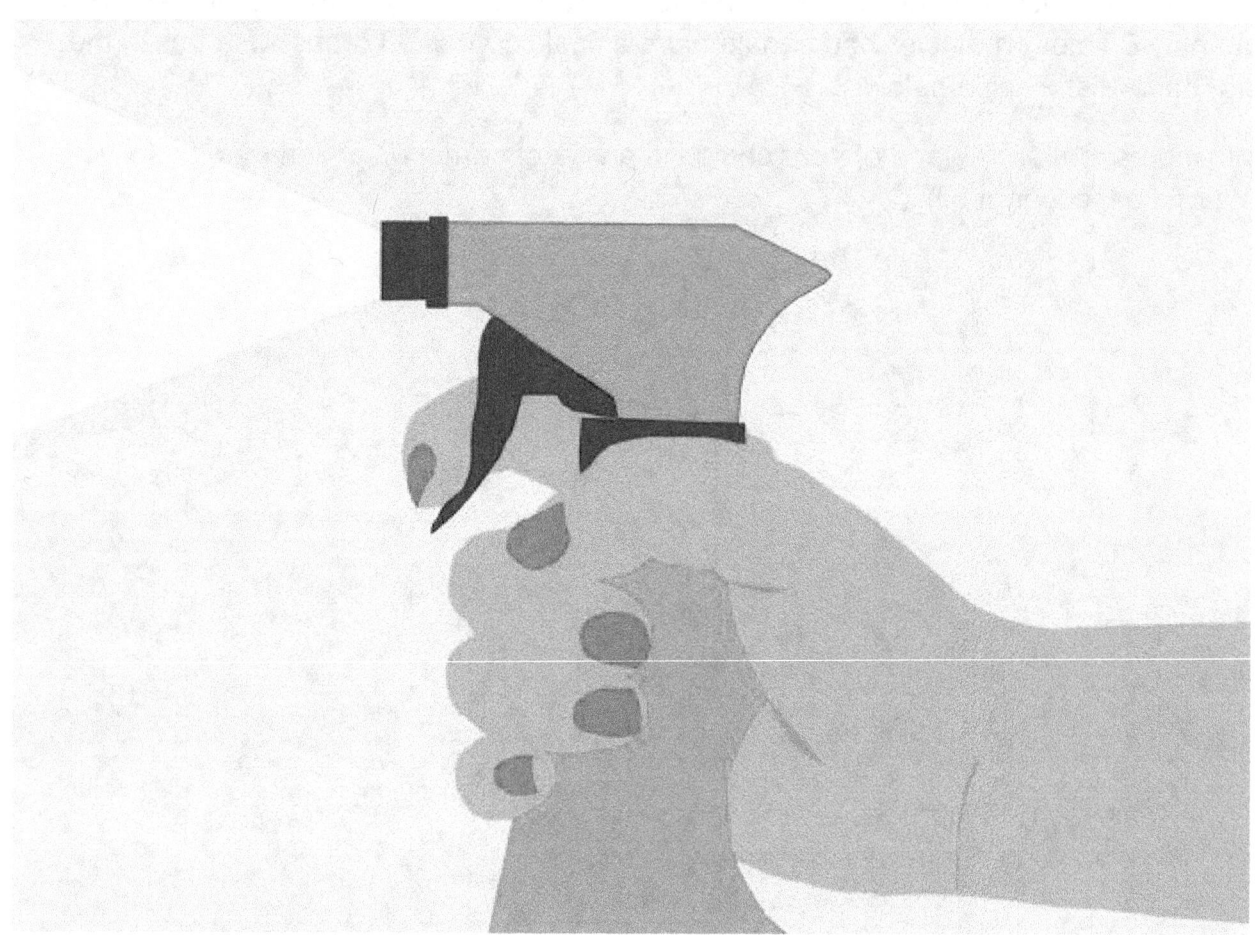

Bath Crystals Recipe

If you want to use your aromatherapy knowledge on bath crystals increase the ingredient quantity of your blend 4 times to what it is. You need 20 drops to make the recipe.

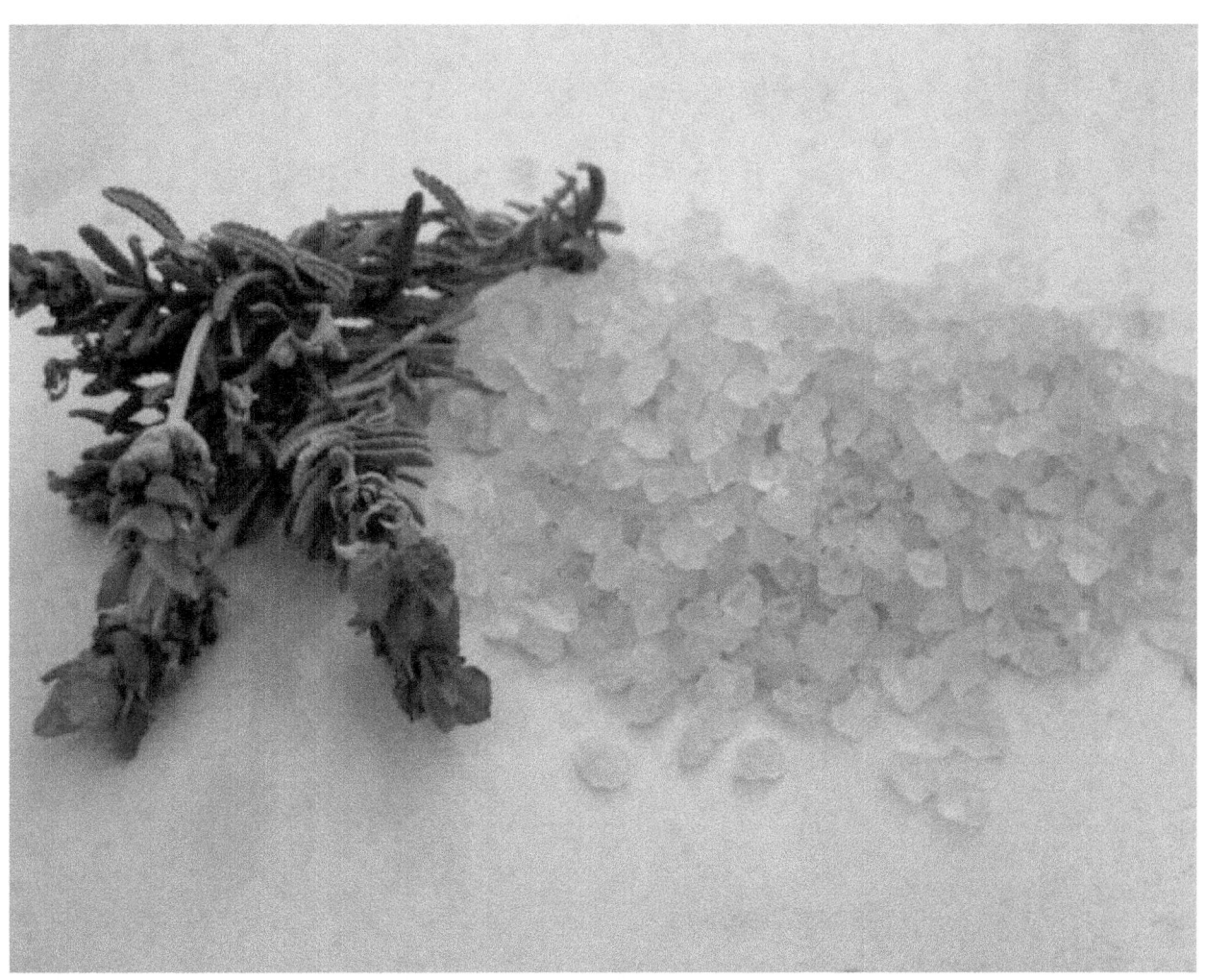

Bath Oil Aroma Recipe

For this you need to multiply the ingredients amount by 3 and make sure they accumulate to at least 15 drops. First add 2 Oz of your chosen carrier oil to your essential oil blend and store this in a sterile bottle. When you are preparing the bath just add in ¼ of your mixture.

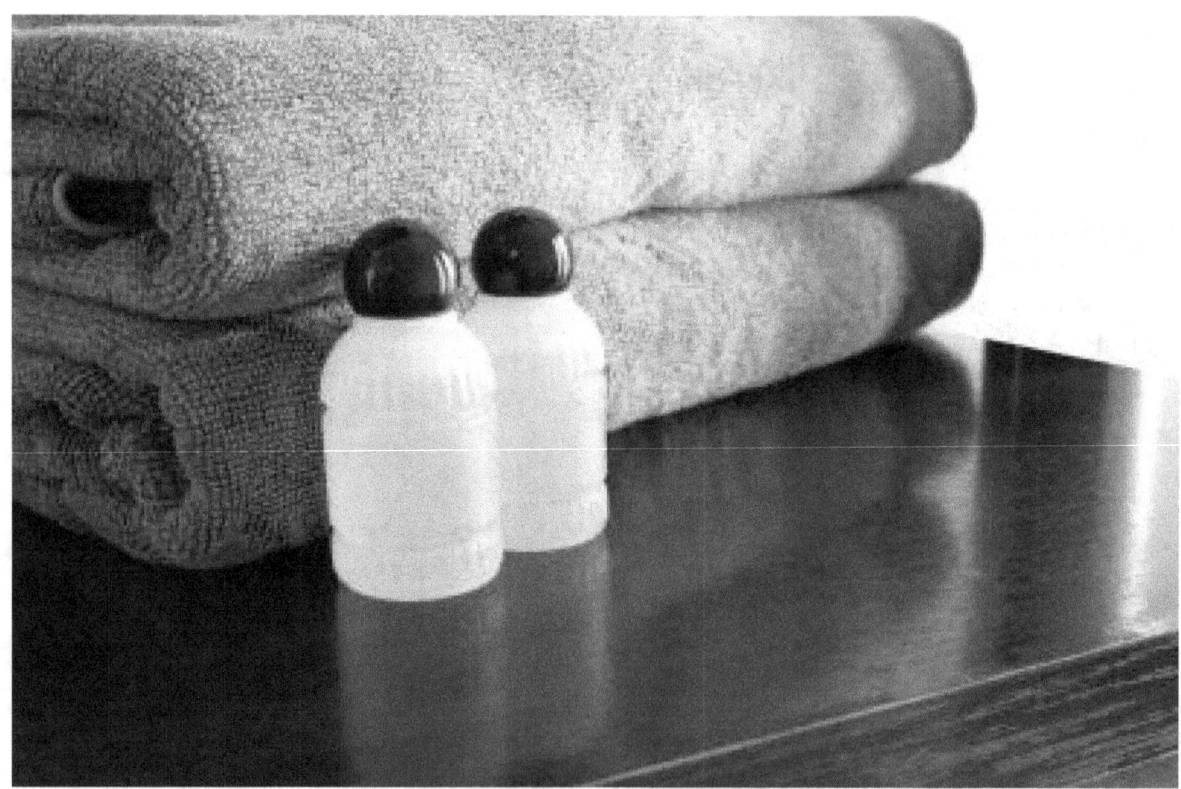

Psychological Well Being

Stress Reduction Blend

Frankincense oil- 1 drop

Geranium Oil- 1 drop

Bergamot Oil- 3 drops

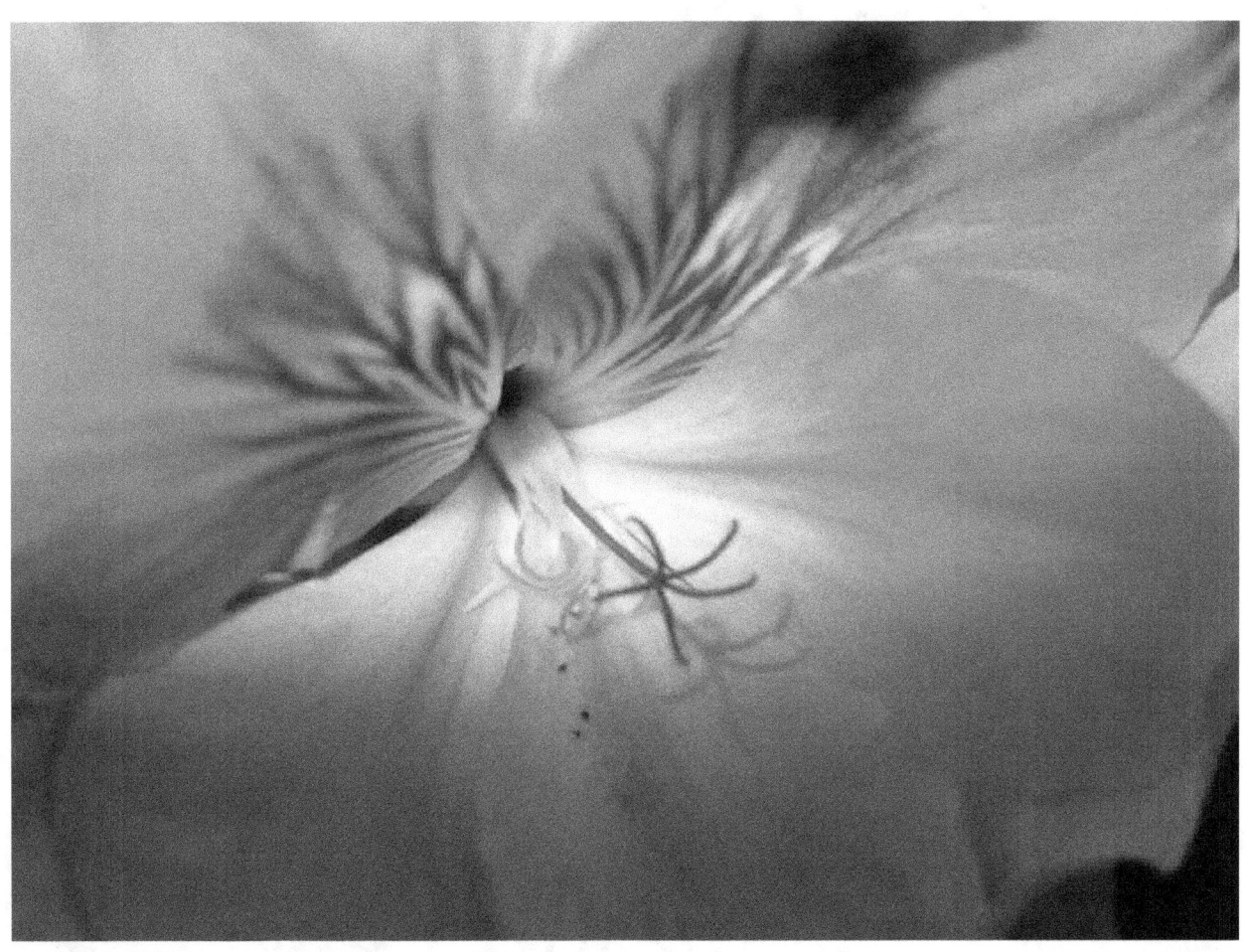

Anger Management Blend

Orange- 2 drops

Bergamot Oil- 2 drops

Roman Chamomile- 2 drops

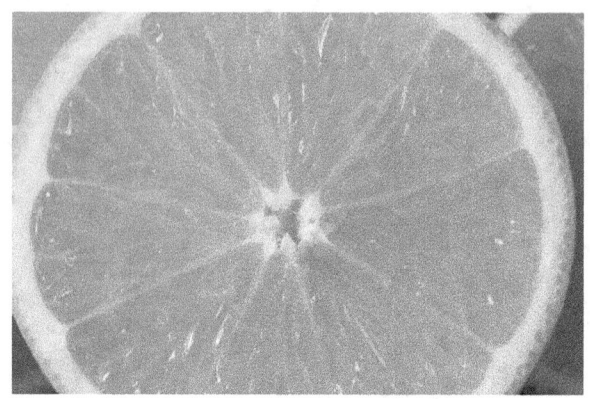

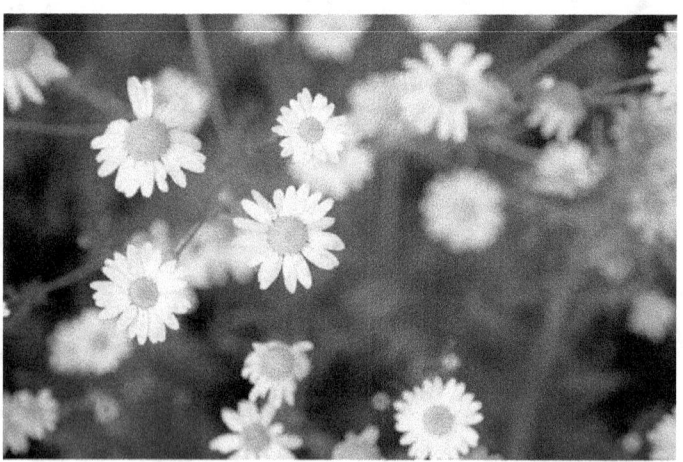

Anxiety Reduction Blend

Vetiver Oil- 1 drop

Mandarin Oil- 2 drops

Lavender Oil- 1 drop

Rose essential oil- 1 drop

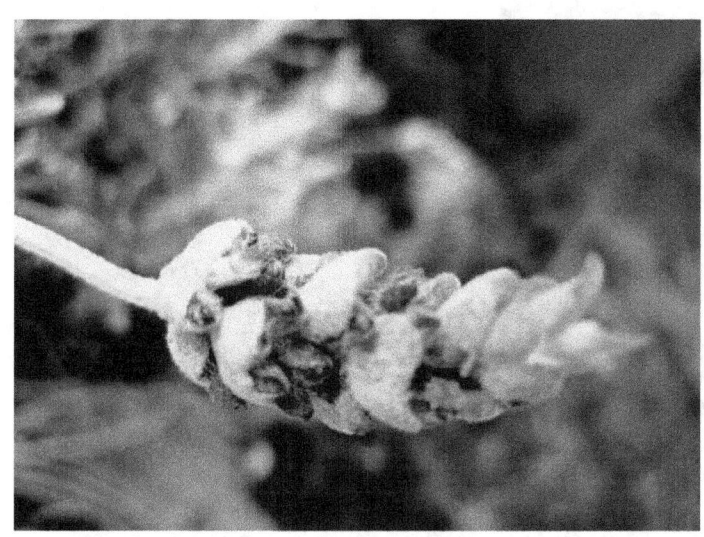

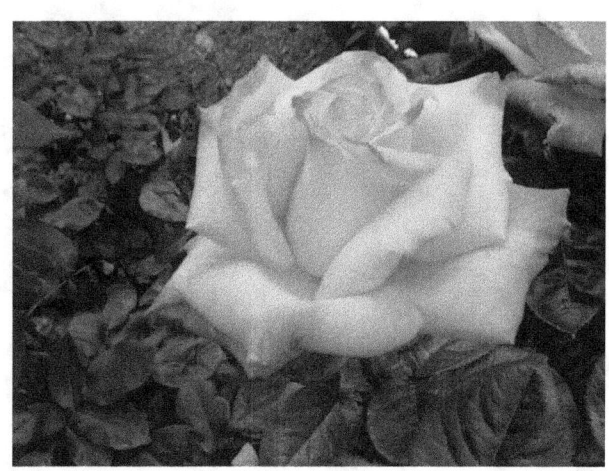

Confidence Boosting Blend

Rosemary Oil- 2 drops

Orange- 3 drops

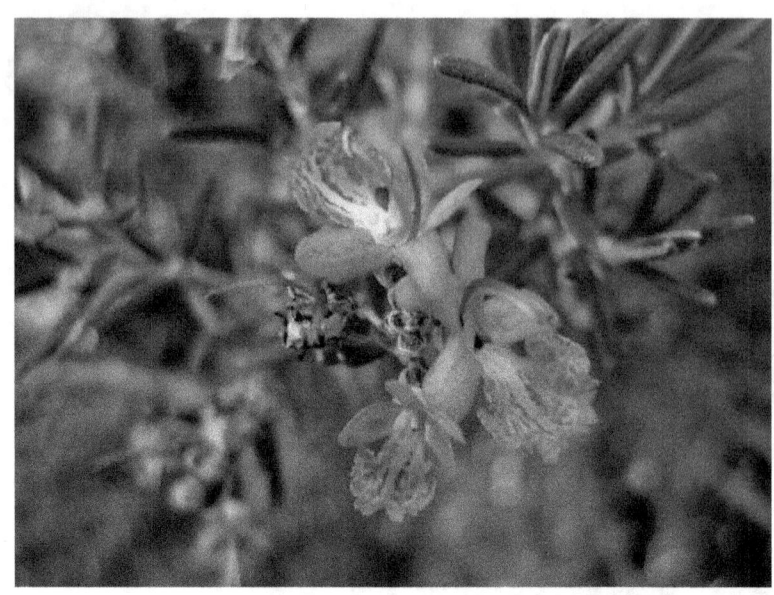

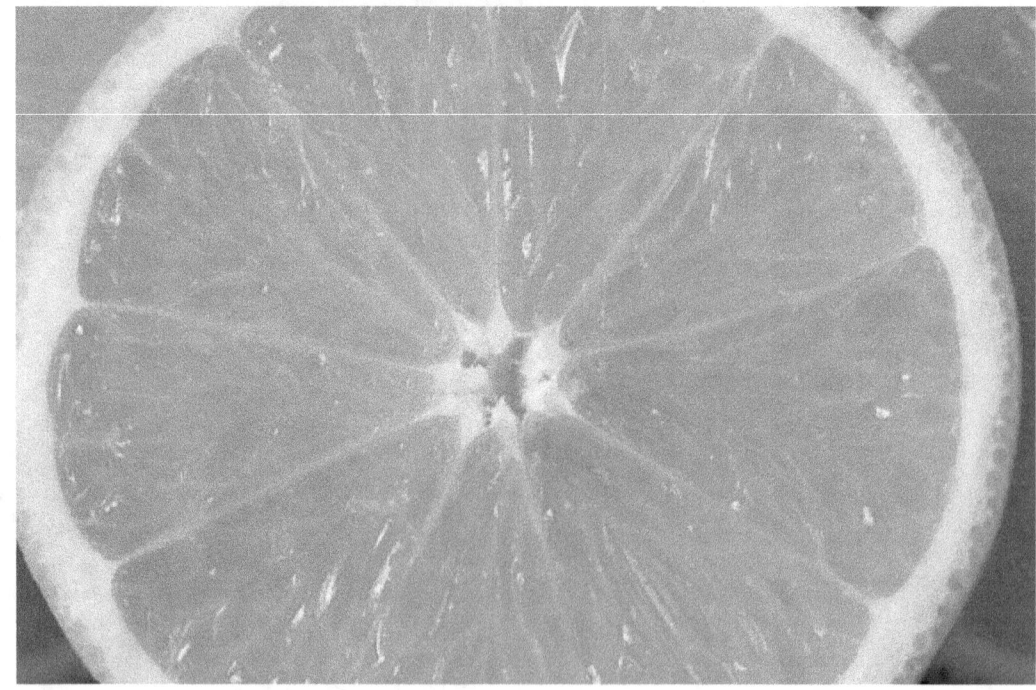

Grief Coping Blend

Sandalwood essential oil- 3 drops

Rose- 1 drop

Neroli- 1 drop

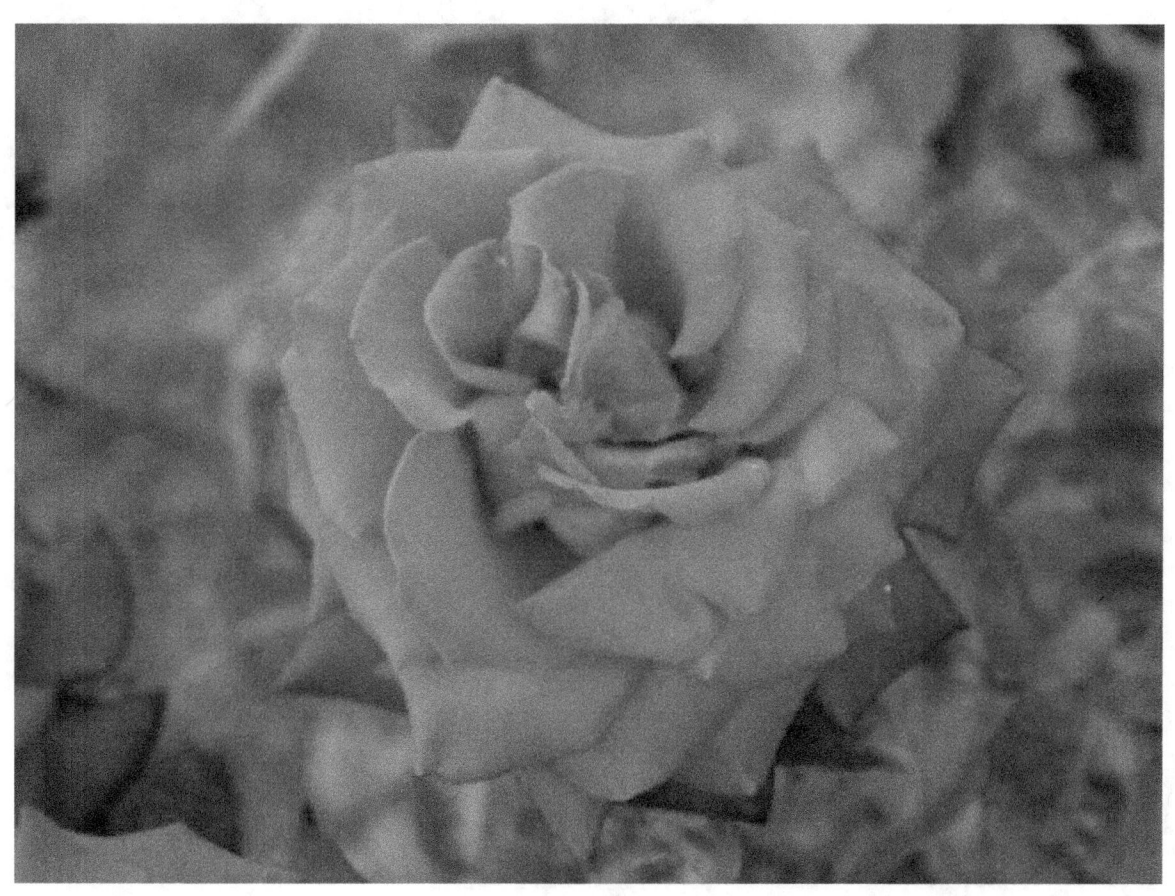

To Reduce Fear and Energize

Vetiver Oil- 1 drop

Roman Chamomile- 2 drops

Clary Sage- 2 drops

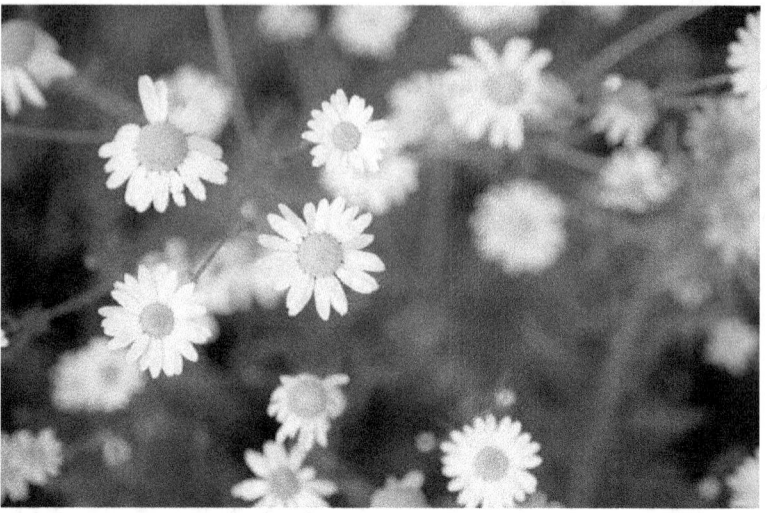

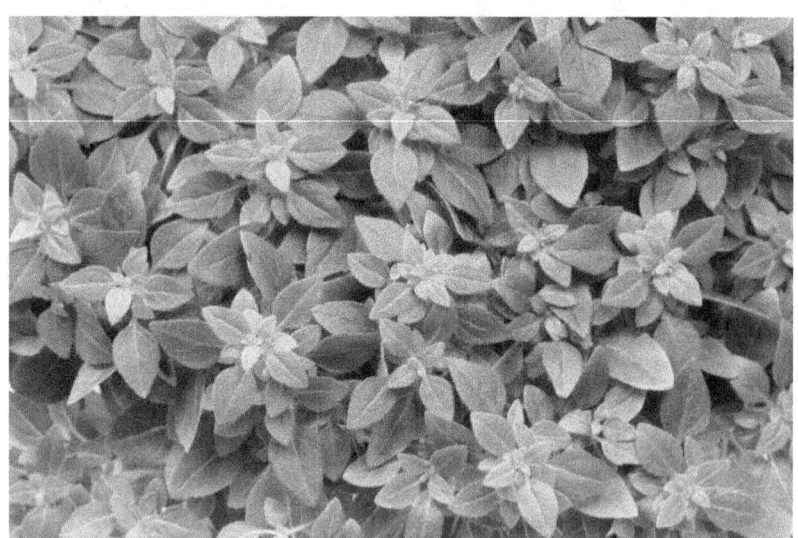

Happiness and Serenity Enhancing Blend

Grapefruit essential oil- 1 drop

Ylang Ylang flower essential oil- 1 drop

Bergamot essential oil- 3 drops

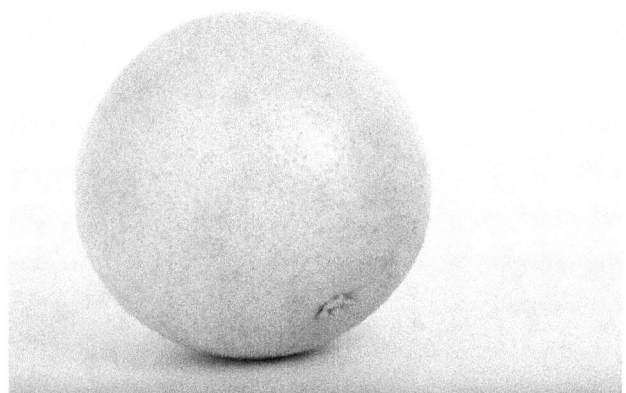

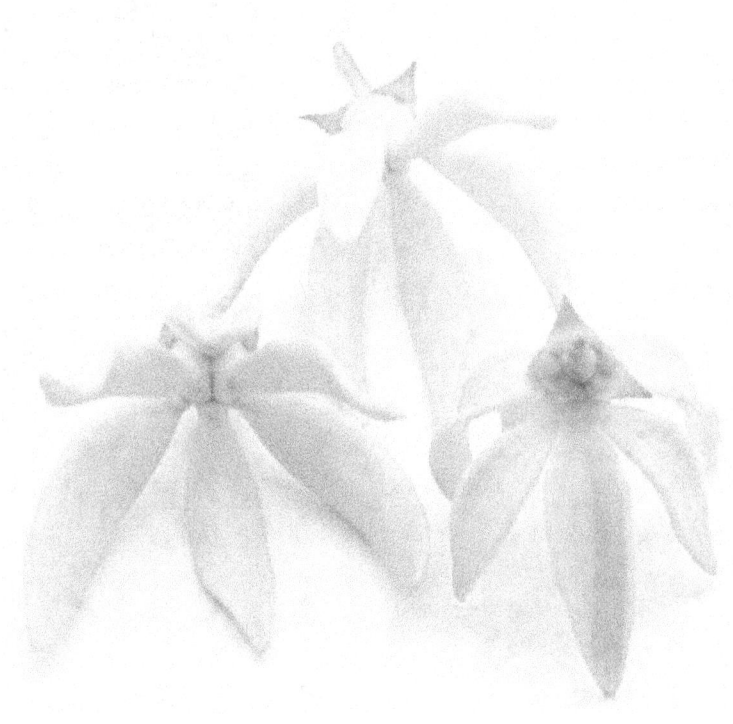

Relaxation Blend

Lavender essential oil- 5 drops

Roman chamomile- 10 drops

Note: For the best calming effect mix this blend into an Oz of carrier oil coconut oil or almond oil and massage on the feet.

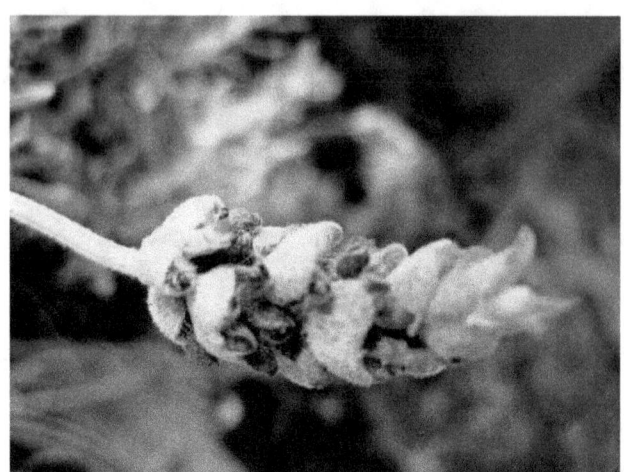

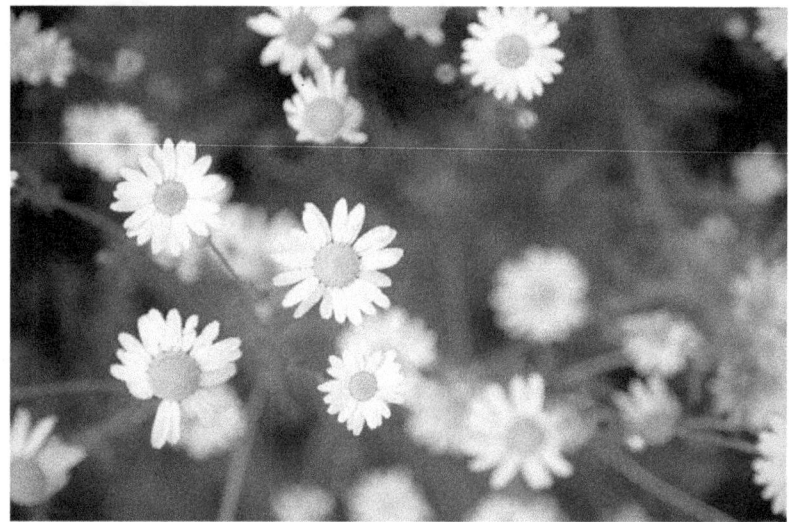

Enhance Memory and Focus

Cypress Oil- 2 drops

Rosemary Oil- 2 drops

Basil- 1 drop

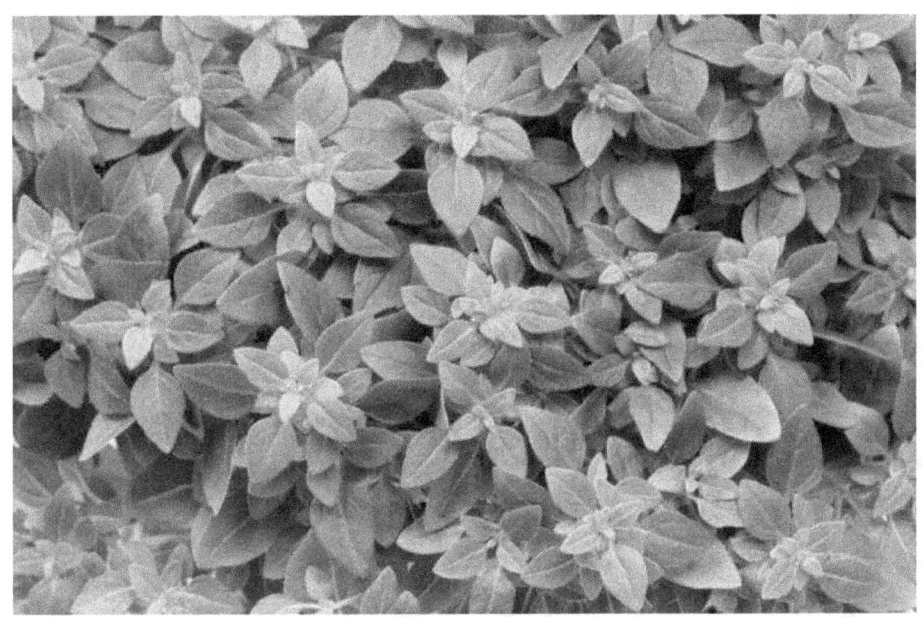

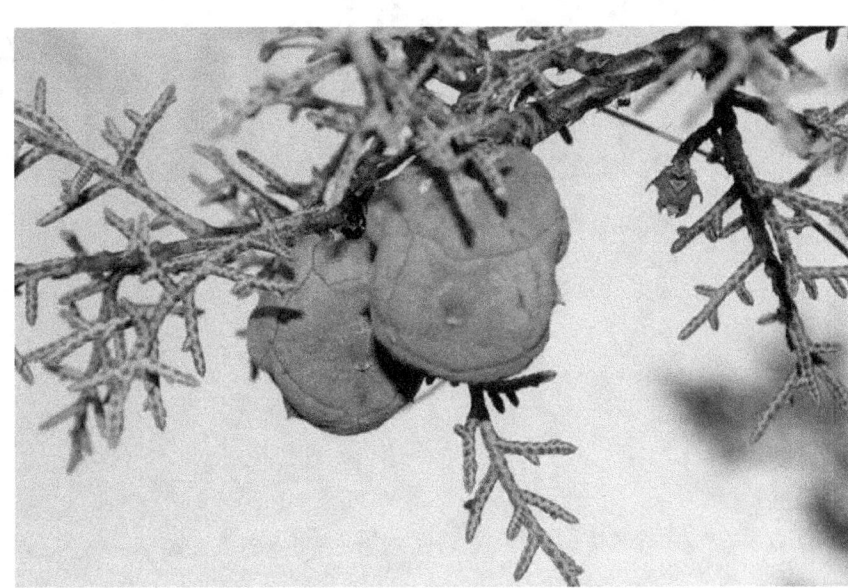

Reduce feelings of Loneliness

Clary Sage- 3 drops

Frankincense- 2 drops

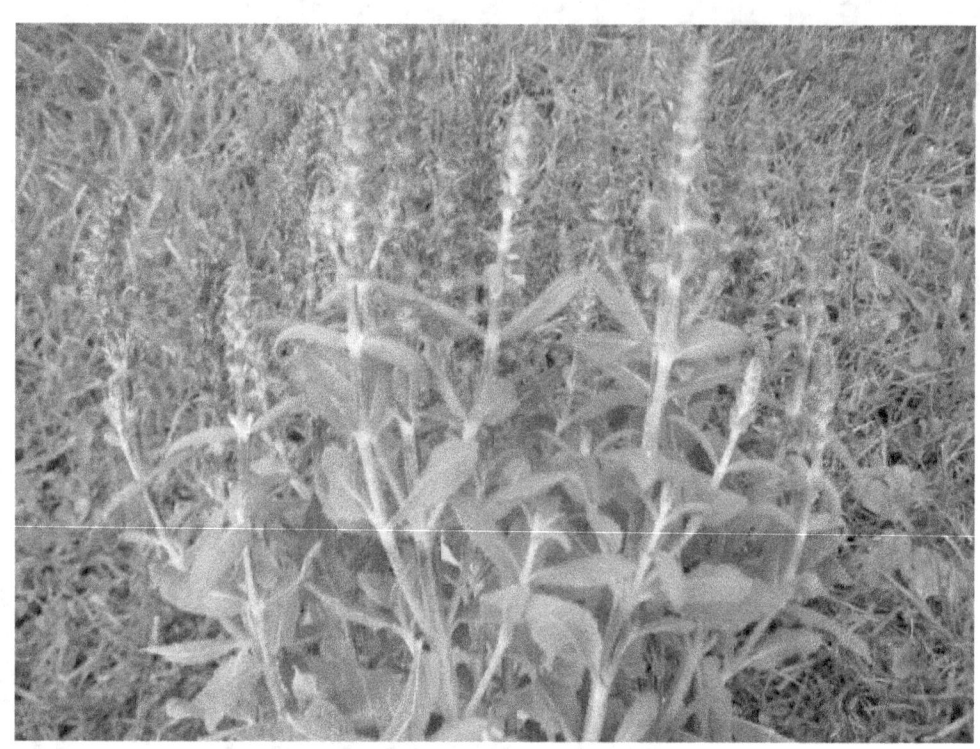

Get Rid Of Irritability

Sandalwood- 4 drops

Neroli- 1 drop

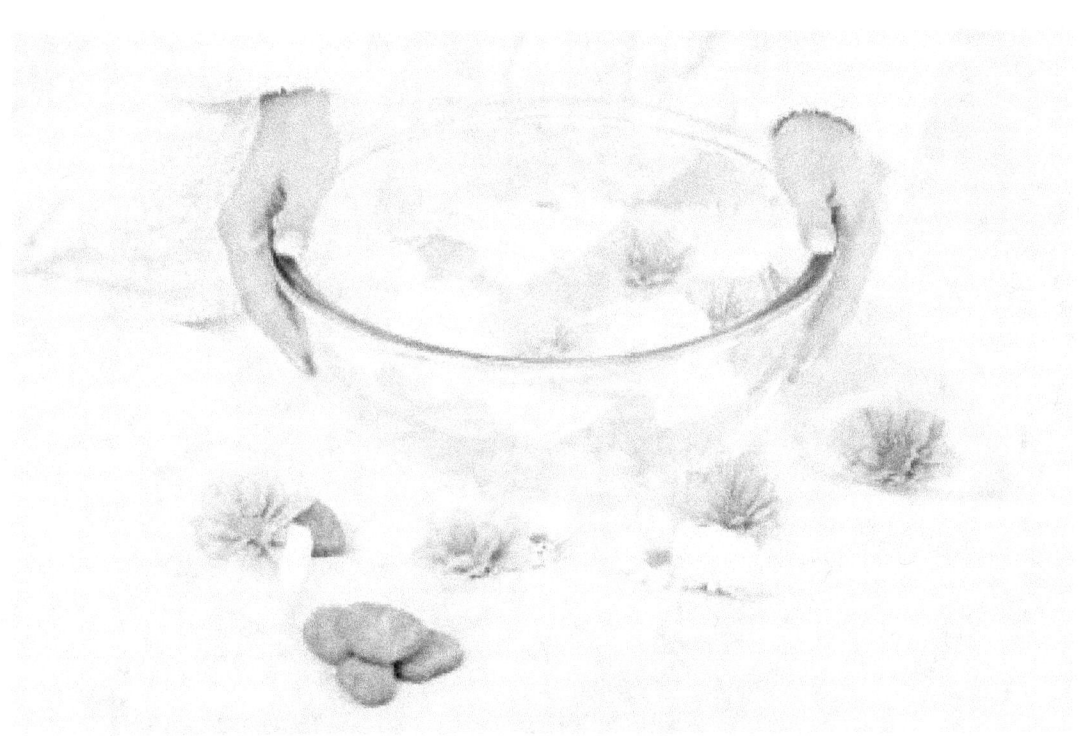

Aromatherapy Know- It- All For Newbies

This book is sectioned out in all the respectful details. However, it's important that we draft out certain tips and suggestions that practitioners wish they knew from the start.

Fragrance Oils Are Not Essential Oils

Perfume oils do not have the same aroma essential oils have so they are not an equal alternative to essential oils in aromatherapy. That being said even if you plan to use aromatherapy for the enjoyment of the aroma you must remember that the benefits of aromatherapy are not gained with perfume oils at all.

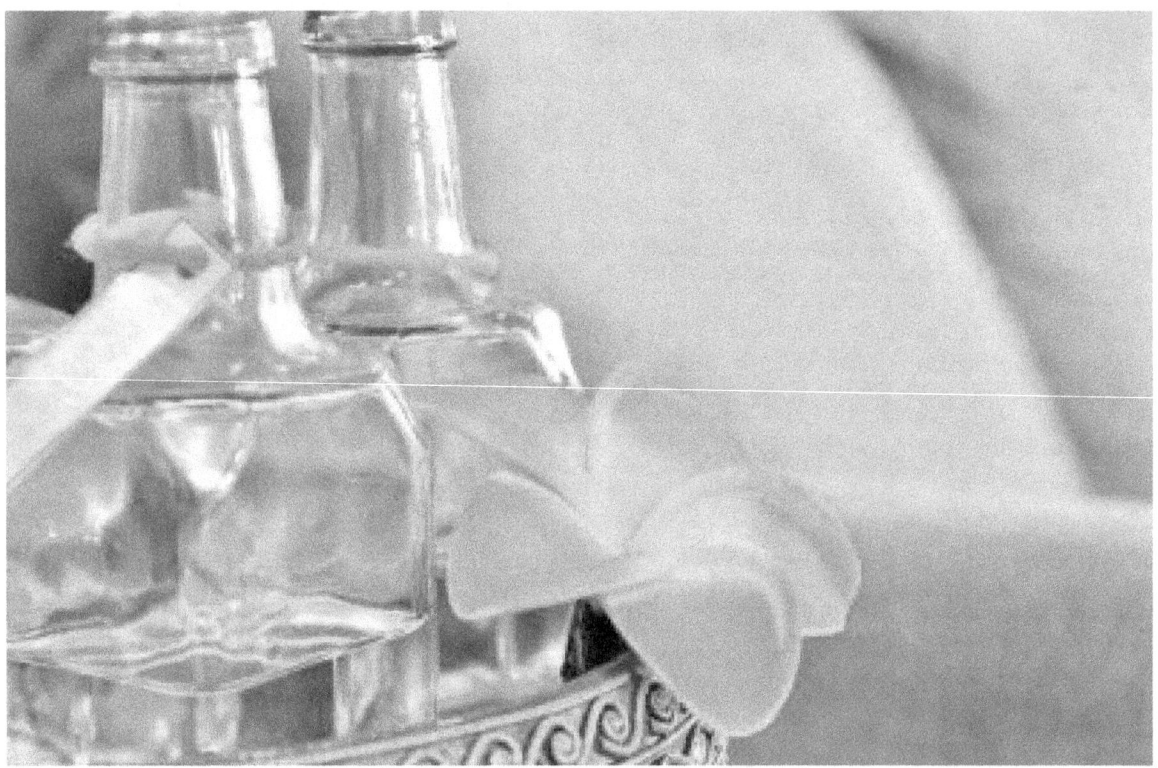

The Rubber Top

One more useful tip to know beforehand is that never make the mistake of buying essential oil bottles that have rubber glass dropper. This leads to the oil turning the cap into gum and that in turn leads to the oil being ruined.

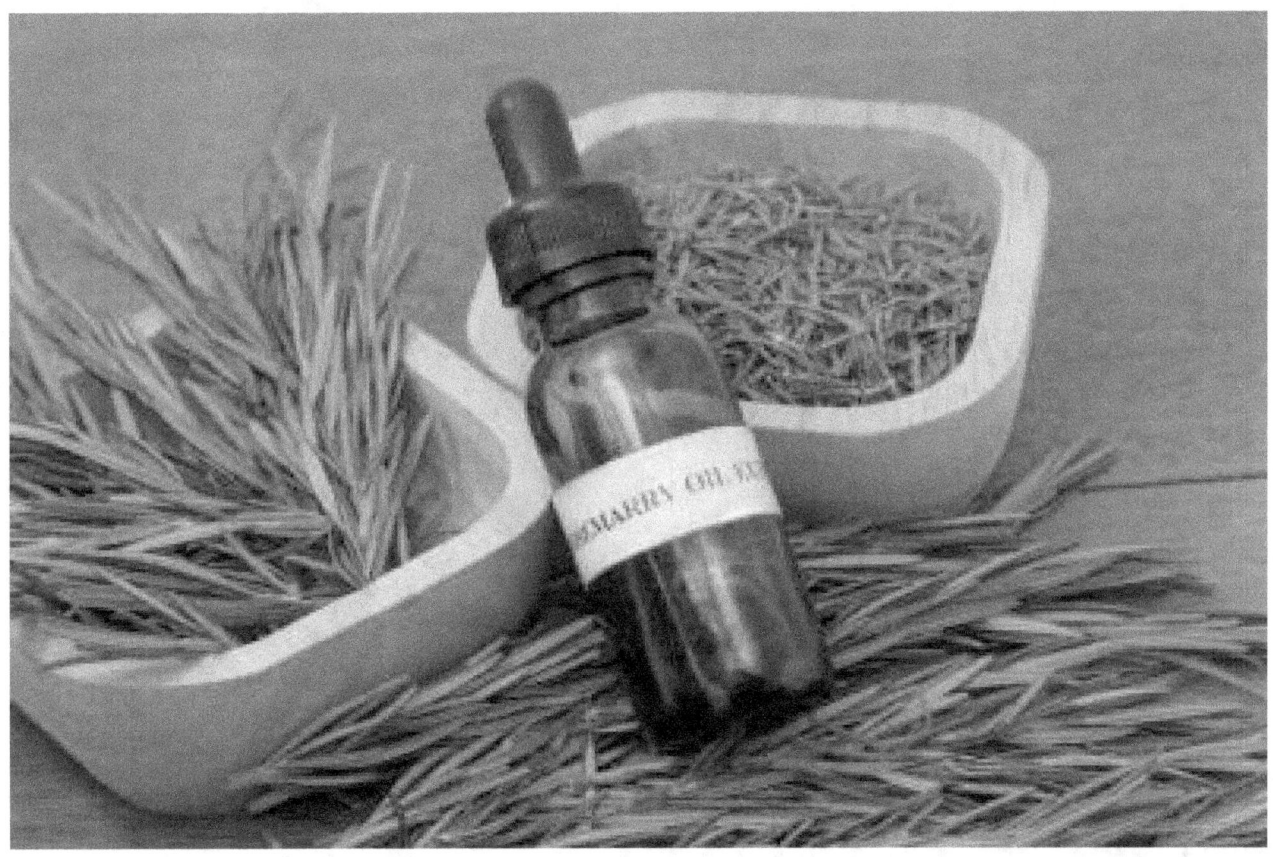

Enlighten Yourself

However it is important that you read and gather as much information as you can on aromatherapy and the profile of all the essential oils that you plan on blending. This book incorporates the safety precautions needed to handle essential oils for aromatherapy however each essential oils come with their own safety precautions which you don't hear about with other oils.

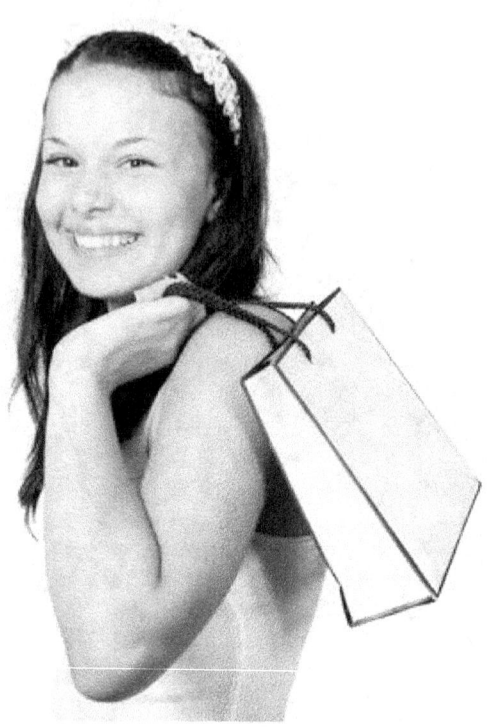

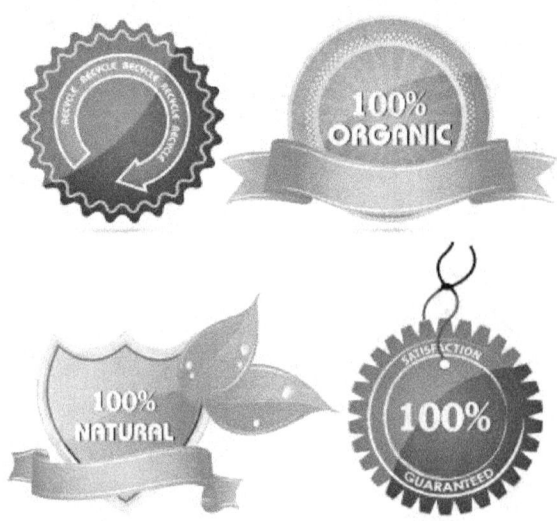

The Right Window Shopping

It a good thing if you are choosy about where you are going to buy the essential oils that you need. The oils quality does vary from label to label plus you need to watch out for companies advertising that their oils are pure and undiluted when they are not.

Learn to compare the oil the same oils that are on offer. Remember, lavender, bay, cedarwood, etc are just names of the plants with which the essential oils are made. You must remind yourself that even among these plants there are several different varieties which lead to several different essential oil extracts. Here, however, you must teach yourself the different botanical names that denote each essential oil's plant.

Another helpful tip is if you remember the country of origin for the oil. Most essential oil sellers will tell you the name of the country of origin as well as the botanical name. You need to take three things into consideration: whether the oils are wildcrafted? Organic? And ethically derived?

Stay Away From No Returns

Steer clear of vendors, street fairs and craft shows. These are limited time affairs and you as a beginner may not be able to exchange a mistaken essential oils. Even if the company is reputable make sure that you have the resources at hand to judge the quality.

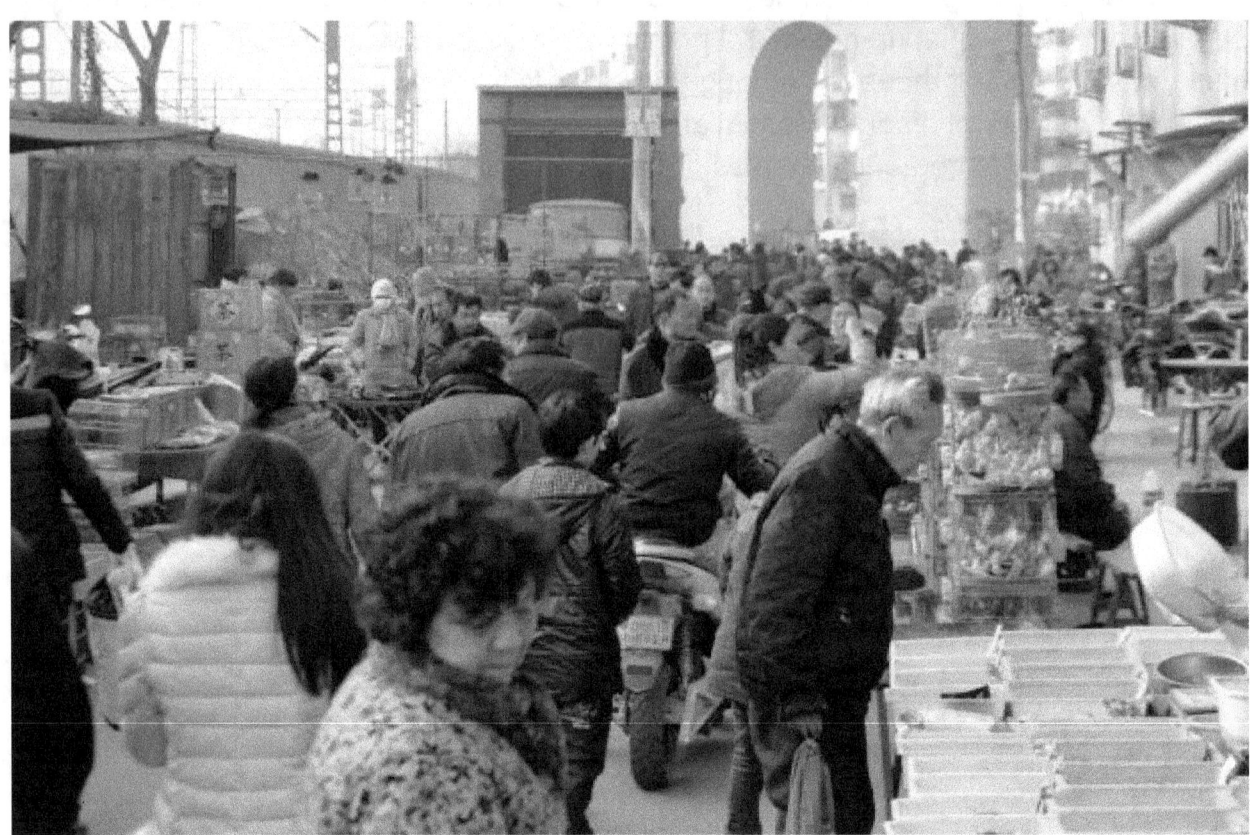

Buy Online

Buying oils from mail orders are always a wise choice. You are given good quality oils at less expensive prices and these are not generic unlike many small health food stores. There is a major difference between

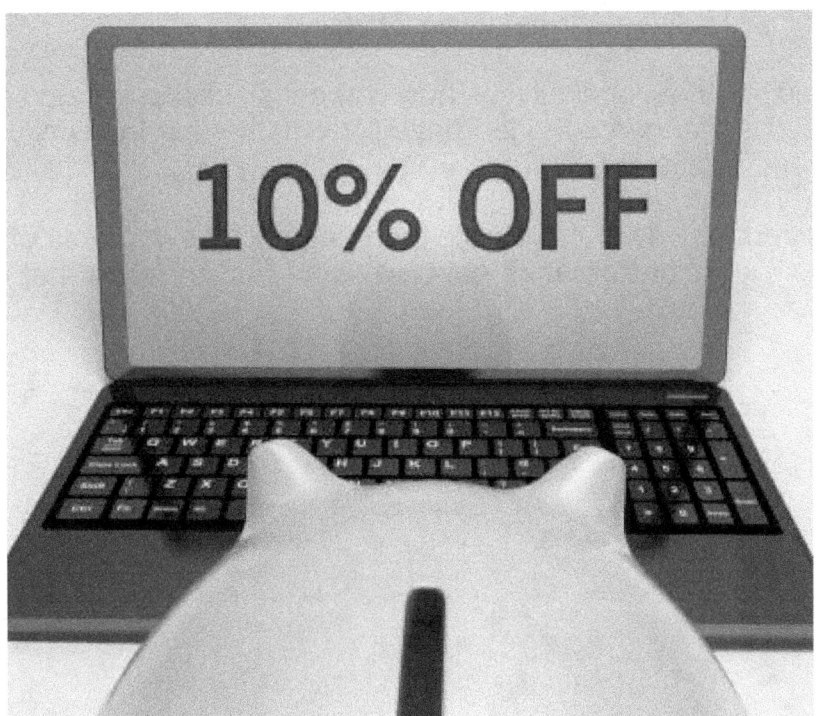

Make sure that you store your oils in a dark glass bottle away from the reach of children. This will make you easily able to distinguish between several different viles. A wise move would be to purchase a wood box holder for all the essential oil boxes

Many people who try aromatherapy for the first time wonder why it never hit the media as aggressively as many other practices have.

Infused oils have been around for years. The name aromatherapy though was coined in the 20th century.

The reason that aromatherapy is fast gaining all the hype today is because the media has been hugely covering all the health conscious trends and somewhere in the middle of that they stumbled upon the term 'aromatherapy' without fully understanding its meaning. Aromatherapy has been here all along it is just that with its increased exposure society is slowly becoming aware of this.

A great example of the popularity is how essential oils are being sold online like everyday goods. This furthered the journey of Aromatherapy Industry's growth and has attracted many enthusiasts too.

Aromatherapy offers an easier solution to many annoying symptoms of everyday stress and low energy. Our ancestors may not have vigorously needed that before but today we do!